DR. LARRY GODSON

Beyond Blemishes

A Comprehensive Guide to Acne-Free Living

Contents

1

Introduction

Welcome to a transformative journey towards clear and healthy skin! This comprehensive guide is designed to empower you with knowledge, practical tips, and effective strategies to achieve radiant and blemish-free skin. Whether you're dealing with acne, navigating the signs of aging, or simply aiming for a vibrant complexion, this guide provides a roadmap for your skincare adventure.

Skincare is not just a routine; it's a holistic approach to self-care and well-being. In the following chapters, we will delve into the fundamentals of skincare, explore the causes of common skin concerns, and equip you with actionable steps to address them. From establishing a daily skincare routine to understanding the role of diet and lifestyle, we'll cover a wide spectrum of topics to guide you towards your skin goals.

Beyond the physical aspects, we'll also explore the emotional impact of skin concerns and provide insights into cultivating a positive relationship with your natural beauty. You'll find practical advice, recommendations for products, and even resources for ongoing support in your skincare journey.

Remember, your skin is unique, and so is your journey. Whether you're starting a skincare routine for the first time or seeking to enhance an existing one, this guide is crafted to be your companion, offering guidance and inspiration at every step.

Let's embark on this journey together — a journey towards clear, radiant, and confident skin. Here's to the glow within you!

2

Understanding Acne

Acne is more than just a skin condition; it's a common concern that affects people of all ages and backgrounds. In this chapter, we'll explore the intricacies of acne, unraveling its origins and understanding the various factors that contribute to its development.

What is Acne?

Acne is a skin disorder characterized by the presence of pimples, blackheads, whiteheads, and, in severe cases, cysts. These blemishes typically appear on the face, neck, chest, back, and shoulders. Understanding the different types of acne, such as comedonal, inflammatory, and cystic acne, is crucial in tailoring an effective treatment plan.

At its core, acne is a multifaceted skin disorder that manifests in various forms, impacting millions of individuals worldwide. It is marked by the presence of different types of skin blemishes, ranging from mild comedones to more severe inflammatory lesions.

Acne, scientifically known as acne vulgaris, is a chronic skin condition that primarily affects the pilosebaceous units—hair follicles and sebaceous glands. These units are found in abundance on the face, neck, chest, back, and shoulders. Acne commonly begins during adolescence but can persist into adulthood, presenting a wide spectrum of manifestations.

The Causes of Acne

Acne doesn't have a single cause; rather, it emerges from a combination of factors. Hormonal fluctuations, excessive oil production, clogged pores, and bacterial overgrowth are key contributors. Environmental factors, genetics, and lifestyle choices also play significant roles in the development and exacerbation of acne.

Acne is a complex skin condition with a multitude of contributing factors. By comprehending the underlying causes, individuals can better tailor their approach to prevention and treatment. In this chapter, we dissect the intricate web of elements that lead to the development of acne.

1. Sebum Overproduction: Balancing Act Gone Awry

The sebaceous glands, responsible for producing sebum (skin oil), play a crucial role in maintaining skin health. However, when these glands go into overdrive, excess sebum can clog hair follicles, initiating the acne cascade.

2. Hair Follicle Blockage: The Foundation of Acne Formation

The constant shedding of dead skin cells is a natural part of skin renewal. Yet, when these cells mix with excess sebum, they create a sticky plug, obstructing the hair follicles. This environment becomes a breeding ground for acne-causing bacteria.

3. Bacterial Activity: Propionibacterium acnes Takes Center Stage

Within the obstructed hair follicles, Propionibacterium acnes (P. acnes) bacteria thrive. As these bacteria multiply, they trigger an inflammatory response from the immune system, leading to the characteristic redness and swelling associated with acne lesions.

4. Hormonal Influences: Androgens and Acne Dynamics

Hormones, particularly androgens, play a pivotal role in acne development. During puberty, increased androgen levels stimulate sebum production. Hormonal fluctuations during menstruation and pregnancy can also influence sebum secretion, making these periods more prone to acne breakouts.

5. Genetics: The Acne Blueprint

Family history can significantly impact an individual's predisposition to acne. Genetic factors influence how the skin responds to hormonal changes, inflammation, and other acne triggers.

6. Dietary Factors: Unmasking the Acne Culprits

While the link between diet and acne is complex and varies among individuals, certain foods may contribute to acne development. High-glycemic foods, dairy products, and certain fats have been studied for their potential impact on acne.

7. Environmental Factors: Unseen Forces at Play

External elements, such as pollution and exposure to certain chemicals, can exacerbate acne. Understanding how environmental factors interact with the skin can guide protective measures.

8. Lifestyle Habits: Stress, Sleep, and Skincare Practices

Stress, lack of sleep, and improper skincare routines can influence acne. Managing stress, prioritizing restful sleep, and adopting effective skincare habits are integral aspects of a holistic acne prevention strategy.

In this chapter, we've peeled back the layers to reveal the intricate dance of factors that contribute to acne. Armed with this knowledge, readers can embark on a more informed journey towards clearer skin, addressing not only the symptoms but also the root causes of this common skin concern.

Different Types of Acne

Not all acne is created equal. This section will delve into the distinct characteristics of various acne types, helping readers identify and understand their specific conditions. From blackheads and whiteheads to papules and nodules, each type requires a tailored approach for effective management.

Acne is a diverse skin condition, presenting in various forms and severities. Recognizing the specific types of acne is crucial for tailoring an effective treatment plan. In this chapter, we'll explore the different manifestations of acne, from non-inflammatory comedones to more severe inflammatory lesions.

1. Non-Inflammatory Acne: Comedones

Blackheads (Open Comedones):

Blackheads occur when hair follicles are clogged with a combination of dead skin cells and sebum. The surface of the clog darkens due to oxidation, giving it a black appearance. Unlike whiteheads, blackheads have an open pore, allowing the material to be exposed to air.

Whiteheads (Closed Comedones):

Whiteheads are similar to blackheads but have a closed pore. The hair follicle is completely blocked, resulting in a small, flesh-colored bump on the skin. These closed comedones may be more resistant to topical treatments.

2. Inflammatory Acne: The Battle Beneath the Surface

Papules:

Papules are small, raised, and often pink or red bumps on the skin. They result from inflammation and infection around the hair follicles. While papules are not filled with pus, they can be tender to the touch.

Pustules:

Pustules are what we commonly refer to as pimples. These are small, round lesions filled with yellow or white pus. Pustules often have a red base and may be surrounded by inflammation.

Nodules:

Nodules are larger, more severe, and deeper than pustules. These solid, painful lumps form beneath the surface of the skin. Nodular acne requires professional treatment and may lead to scarring.

Cysts:

Cystic acne is the most severe form of acne. Cysts are large, painful, pus-filled lesions that extend deep into the skin. Cystic acne often causes significant inflammation and can result in long-term scarring.

Understanding the distinctions between these types of acne is crucial for developing an effective treatment strategy. In the following chapters, we'll explore various approaches, from daily skincare routines to professional treatments, designed to address each type of acne and promote clearer, healthier skin.

The Emotional Impact of Acne

Acne's impact extends beyond the physical realm; it can take a toll on emotional well-being and self-esteem. We'll explore the psychological aspects of living with acne, offering insights into coping strategies and building resilience. Understanding the emotional dimensions of acne is a crucial step towards achieving not just clear skin but a positive self-image.

1. **The Visible Burden: Acne's Impact on Self-Esteem**

Acne's visibility can lead to a significant impact on self-esteem. Individuals may experience feelings of embarrassment, shame, and self-consciousness, especially during acne flare-ups. The perception of acne as a flaw can take a toll on one's self-image.

2. Social and Peer Dynamics: Navigating Relationships

Social interactions, particularly during adolescence, can be challenging for those with acne. Fear of judgment, teasing, or bullying may lead to social withdrawal. This chapter explores strategies for building confidence and maintaining social connections despite the challenges posed by acne.

3. The Psychological Toll: Anxiety and Depression

Living with persistent acne can contribute to heightened levels of anxiety and, in some cases, depression. Coping with the emotional distress associated with acne requires a holistic approach that addresses both the physical and emotional aspects of this skin condition.

4. Empowerment Through Self-Care: Building Resilience

Acknowledging the emotional impact of acne is the first step toward building resilience. This section explores self-care practices, mindfulness techniques, and therapeutic approaches that can empower individuals to navigate the emotional challenges associated with acne.

5. Seeking Support: Connecting with Others

Sharing experiences and seeking support from friends, family, or support groups can be instrumental in managing the emotional toll of acne. This chapter provides guidance on effective communication and encourages open dialogue about the emotional impact of acne.

6. Professional Help: Mental Health Support

For individuals facing significant emotional distress, seeking professional mental health support is a crucial step. This section discusses the role of therapists, counselors, and mental health professionals in providing guidance and coping strategies.

By addressing the emotional impact of acne, this chapter aims to equip readers with tools to foster self-acceptance, resilience, and a positive mindset. Clearing the path to emotional well-being is an integral part of the journey to achieving not just clear skin but a healthier, more confident sense of self.

Understanding acne involves recognizing its diverse forms, understanding its underlying causes, and appreciating the unique factors that contribute to individual experiences. As we embark on this exploration, we aim to empower readers with knowledge to effectively address and manage this common skin concern.

3

Skincare Basics

In the pursuit of acne-free skin, establishing a solid skincare routine is fundamental. This chapter explores the essential components of a daily skincare regimen, from proper cleansing techniques to the importance of sun protection.

Daily Skincare Routine

A consistent and effective daily skincare routine is key to managing and preventing acne. This section will guide you through the essential steps of a basic skincare regimen designed to promote clear, healthy skin.

1. **Cleansing: The First Step to Clear Skin**
   Effective cleansing is the cornerstone of a good skincare routine. This section provides insights into choosing the right cleanser based on skin type, the importance of gentle cleansing, and the proper technique for removing impurities without exacerbating acne

Understanding Your Skin Type:
   Before choosing a cleanser, it's crucial to identify your skin type. Whether you have oily, dry, combination, or sensitive skin will influence the type of

cleanser that works best for you.

Selecting a Gentle Cleanser:

Opt for a mild, non-comedogenic cleanser that won't strip your skin of essential oils. Look for ingredients like salicylic acid or benzoyl peroxide for their acne-fighting properties.

Proper Cleansing Technique:

Gently massage the cleanser onto damp skin using circular motions, then rinse thoroughly with lukewarm water. Avoid harsh scrubbing, as it can irritate the skin and exacerbate acne.

2. Toning: Balancing Your Skin

Toning helps balance the skin's pH and prepares it for subsequent skincare products. Readers will learn about the benefits of toners, including their role in removing residual cleanser, minimizing pores, and providing a refreshing base for further treatments.

Toning Benefits:

Toners help balance your skin's pH levels, remove any remaining traces of cleanser, and prepare your skin to absorb subsequent products more effectively. Look for alcohol-free toners to avoid excessive dryness.

Application Tips:

Apply toner using a cotton pad or your fingertips, gently patting it onto your skin. Focus on areas prone to acne but avoid the eye area. Toners with ingredients like witch hazel or niacinamide can be beneficial for acne-prone skin.

3. Moisturizing: Hydration for All Skin Types

Contrary to common misconceptions, even oily or acne-prone skin needs hydration. This section explores the importance of moisturizing, the types of moisturizers suitable for different skin types, and how to maintain a proper moisture balance without clogging pores.

Importance of Moisturizing:
Even if you have oily or acne-prone skin, moisturizing is essential. It helps maintain the skin's barrier function and prevents overproduction of oil as a compensatory mechanism.

Choosing the Right Moisturizer:
Select a non-comedogenic, oil-free moisturizer. Ingredients like hyaluronic acid or glycerin can provide hydration without clogging pores. Apply the moisturizer while your skin is still damp to lock in moisture.

Incorporating these three steps into your daily routine provides a solid foundation for healthy skin. In the following sections, we'll explore additional steps, such as targeted treatments and sun protection, to enhance your skincare regimen and address specific acne concerns.

Choosing the Right Products

Navigating the world of skincare products can be overwhelming, but understanding your skin's needs and the purpose of different ingredients can empower you to make informed choices. This section will guide you through the process of selecting products tailored to your skin type and concerns.

1. Understanding Ingredients: Deciphering Product Labels
Navigating the world of skincare products can be daunting. This section provides a guide to deciphering product labels, recognizing beneficial ingredients, and identifying potential irritants. Readers will gain the knowledge needed to make informed choices when selecting skincare products

Identifying Beneficial Ingredients:
Look for key ingredients known for their positive effects on the skin. For acne-prone skin, ingredients like salicylic acid, benzoyl peroxide, niacinamide, and hyaluronic acid can be beneficial. Be cautious of harsh ingredients like alcohol, which can cause irritation.

Avoiding Potential Irritants:
If you have sensitive skin, avoid products containing fragrances, dyes, or alcohol. These can trigger irritation and worsen acne symptoms. Opt for products labeled as "fragrance-free" or "non-comedogenic."

2. Tailoring Products to Skin Type: Customizing Your Routine

Every individual's skin is unique, and the right products depend on specific needs. This part of the chapter outlines skincare routines for various skin types, including tips for those with sensitive, oily, dry, or combination skin.

Products for Oily Skin:
For those with oily skin, lightweight, oil-free formulations work best. Consider gel-based cleansers, oil-free moisturizers, and products with ingredients like salicylic acid to control excess oil.

Products for Dry Skin:
Dry skin requires hydrating products. Look for creamy cleansers, moisturizers with ingredients like hyaluronic acid, and gentle exfoliants to remove dry, flaky skin without causing irritation.

Combination Skin Solutions:
If you have a combination of oily and dry areas, customize your routine by using products formulated for each specific area. This may include a gentle cleanser for the entire face and a more hydrating moisturizer for dry areas.

Understanding your skin's unique needs is essential for selecting products that will contribute to its overall health. In the next section, we'll explore the importance of sun protection and how to choose a sunscreen that complements your skincare routine, ensuring comprehensive care for your skin.

Sun Protection

Protecting your skin from the harmful effects of the sun is a non-negotiable aspect of any skincare routine. In this section, we'll explore the importance of sunscreen and provide guidance on choosing the right product to safeguard your skin from sun damage.

1. **Importance of Sunscreen: Defending Your Skin**

Sun protection is non-negotiable in any skincare routine. This section emphasizes the role of sunscreen in preventing sun damage, premature aging, and hyperpigmentation. Special attention is given to selecting sunscreens suitable for acne-prone skin.

Understanding UV Rays:

The sun emits ultraviolet (UV) rays, which can damage your skin and contribute to premature aging, hyperpigmentation, and an increased risk of skin cancer. Sunscreen acts as a shield, blocking or absorbing these harmful rays.

Daily Use:

Sunscreen is not just for sunny days; it should be a daily habit, even on cloudy or winter days. UV rays can penetrate clouds and cause damage even when the sun isn't visibly strong.

2. **Incorporating Sunscreen into Daily Life: Tips for Application**

Many individuals struggle with consistent sunscreen use. This part offers practical tips on seamlessly integrating sunscreen into daily routines and dispels common myths surrounding its application.

Choosing the Right Sunscreen:

Select a broad-spectrum sunscreen with at least SPF 30. For acne-prone skin, opt for oil-free, non-comedogenic formulations. Look for ingredients like zinc oxide or titanium dioxide, which are less likely to clog pores.

Application Tips:

Apply sunscreen generously to all exposed skin, including your face, neck, and ears. Don't forget often overlooked areas like the back of your hands. Reapply every two hours, more frequently if you're sweating or swimming.

Makeup with SPF:

Consider using makeup with built-in sun protection, but don't rely solely on it. Apply a dedicated sunscreen underneath for comprehensive protection.

Protecting your skin from the sun is a proactive step in maintaining its health and preventing premature aging.

4

Nutrition and Acne

A holistic approach to acne management involves not only external skincare but also internal care through nutrition. This chapter explores the intricate relationship between diet and acne, providing insights into foods that may exacerbate or alleviate symptoms.

The Role of Diet in Acne

Understanding the connection between diet and acne is a crucial step in adopting a holistic approach to skincare. This section explores the intricate relationship between the foods we consume, hormonal balance, and skin health

Understanding the Connection:

Research suggests that certain dietary factors can influence the development and severity of acne. This section delves into the complex interplay between diet, hormones, and skin health.

Complex Interplay:

The impact of diet on acne involves a complex interplay of various factors. Hormonal fluctuations, inflammation, and the production of sebum, the skin's natural oil, can all be influenced by the foods we eat.

Hormonal Changes:

Certain foods can affect hormone levels, particularly insulin-like growth factor 1 (IGF-1) and insulin. Elevated insulin levels may stimulate the production of sebum, contributing to the development of acne lesions.

Impact of High-Glycemic Foods:

Foods with a high glycemic index, such as sugary snacks and refined carbohydrates, can spike blood sugar levels, triggering hormonal changes that may contribute to acne. Learn how to make mindful choices to maintain stable blood sugar levels.

Blood Sugar Spikes:

Foods with a high glycemic index, such as sugary snacks, white bread, and other refined carbohydrates, can lead to rapid spikes in blood sugar levels. This spike triggers an insulin response, potentially exacerbating acne by influencing oil production and increasing inflammation.

Hormonal Response:

High-glycemic foods not only impact blood sugar levels but also stimulate the release of hormones like insulin. These hormonal fluctuations can contribute to an environment conducive to acne development.

Understanding the connection between diet and acne is a crucial step in adopting a holistic approach to skincare. This section explores the intricate relationship between the foods we consume, hormonal balance, and skin health.

Foods to Avoid

While dietary influences on acne can vary from person to person, certain foods are commonly associated with exacerbating acne symptoms. This section explores categories of foods that individuals may consider limiting or avoiding to support clearer skin.

Processed Foods: Culprits of Inflammation

Highly processed foods often contain additives and preservatives that may contribute to inflammation. Limiting the consumption of processed snacks and meals can positively impact skin health.

Additives and Preservatives:

Highly processed foods often contain additives, preservatives, and artificial ingredients that may contribute to inflammation. Limiting the intake of packaged snacks and meals can promote skin health.

Fast Food and Fried Treats:

Fast food and fried items, often high in unhealthy fats and processed components, may contribute to skin inflammation. Reducing the frequency of such foods can positively impact acne-prone skin.

Dairy Products: Assessing Your Tolerance

Potential Hormonal Influence:

Some studies suggest a potential link between dairy consumption and acne, possibly due to hormones present in certain dairy products. Individuals may consider exploring dairy alternatives and monitoring their skin's response.

Moderation and Observation:

Moderation is key, and not everyone will experience acne flare-ups from dairy. If you suspect a connection, try reducing or eliminating dairy for a period and observe changes in your skin.

Sugar and Sweets: Managing Sweet Cravings

Increased Insulin Levels:

Excessive sugar intake can lead to increased insulin levels, potentially contributing to inflammation and acne development. Managing sugar intake is crucial for maintaining stable blood sugar levels.

Healthy Alternatives:

Explore healthier alternatives to satisfy sweet cravings, such as fresh fruits, dark chocolate in moderation, or desserts sweetened with natural alternatives like honey or maple syrup.

Making mindful choices about the foods you consume can positively impact your skin's health. In the next section, we'll explore foods to include in your diet, offering a balanced and holistic approach to nutrition for clearer and healthier skin.

Foods to Include

A balanced and nutrient-rich diet is essential for supporting overall health, including the health of your skin. This section explores foods that are beneficial for maintaining clear and healthy skin, providing key nutrients that can contribute to acne prevention.

Antioxidant-Rich Foods: Fighting Oxidative Stress

Antioxidants help combat oxidative stress, which can contribute to inflammation. Incorporate colorful fruits and vegetables, rich in vitamins A, C, and E, into your diet.

Colorful Fruits and Vegetables:

Include a variety of colorful fruits and vegetables in your diet. These foods are rich in antioxidants, such as vitamins A, C, and E, which help combat oxidative stress and inflammation in the body.

Berries:

Berries, including blueberries, strawberries, and raspberries, are particularly high in antioxidants. They can be enjoyed as snacks, added to smoothies, or incorporated into meals.

Omega-3 Fatty Acids: Anti-Inflammatory Power

Foods like fatty fish, flaxseeds, and walnuts provide omega-3 fatty acids, which have anti-inflammatory properties. Learn how these essential fats can support overall skin health.

Fatty Fish:

Include fatty fish in your diet, such as salmon, mackerel, and sardines. These fish are rich in omega-3 fatty acids, which have anti-inflammatory properties that can benefit the skin.

Flaxseeds and Walnuts:

For those who prefer plant-based sources, flaxseeds and walnuts are excellent options. Add them to salads, yogurt, or oatmeal to increase your omega-3 intake.

Hydration: Water for Radiant Skin

Proper hydration is fundamental for skin health. Explore the benefits of drinking an adequate amount of water daily and how it contributes to a clear complexion.

Importance of Water:

Proper hydration is fundamental for skin health. Water helps flush out toxins from the body and supports overall cellular function. Aim to drink an adequate amount of water throughout the day.

Herbal Teas:

Incorporate herbal teas into your routine, such as chamomile or green tea. These teas not only contribute to hydration but also offer potential skin-soothing benefits.

Incorporating these foods into your diet provides essential nutrients that can contribute to healthier skin. In the next section, we'll delve into the importance of hydration and explore practical tips for maintaining proper water intake for radiant and clear skin.

The Importance of Hydration

Proper hydration is not only crucial for overall health but plays a significant role in maintaining clear and radiant skin. This section explores the importance of hydration and provides practical tips for ensuring you stay well-hydrated for optimal skin health.

Water and Skin Health: The Dynamic Connection

Dehydration can affect the skin's elasticity and overall health. Discover the significance of staying well-hydrated for a radiant complexion and learn practical tips for increasing your water intake.

Skin Elasticity:

Adequate hydration contributes to the skin's elasticity, promoting a supple and youthful appearance. Well-hydrated skin is less prone to dryness, flakiness, and irritation.

Toxin Elimination:

Water is essential for the body's natural detoxification process. Proper hydration helps flush out toxins and waste products, reducing the burden on your skin and other organs.

Practical Tips for Hydration: Making it a Habit

Daily Water Intake:
Ensure you're drinking a sufficient amount of water each day. The general recommendation is around eight 8-ounce glasses, but individual needs may vary based on factors such as age, activity level, and climate.

Carry a Water Bottle:
Keep a reusable water bottle with you throughout the day. Having water readily available makes it easier to stay hydrated, especially if you have a busy schedule.

Herbal Teas and Infusions: Hydration with Flavor
Explore herbal teas and infusions that not only contribute to hydration but also offer potential skin-soothing benefits. From chamomile to green tea, discover beverages that can complement your acne management routine.

Hydrating Beverages:
In addition to water, herbal teas and infusions contribute to your overall hydration. Opt for caffeine-free options, and consider teas with skin-friendly ingredients like chamomile or green tea.

Infused Water:
Enhance the flavor of your water by infusing it with slices of fruits, vegetables, or herbs. This adds a refreshing twist and encourages you to drink more water.

By prioritizing hydration as part of your daily routine, you support not only your overall health but also the health and appearance of your skin. In the following chapters, we'll explore additional lifestyle changes, holistic approaches, and skincare practices to further enhance your journey to acne-free living.

5

Lifestyle Changes

Achieving and maintaining clear skin involves not only a robust skincare routine and a balanced diet but also certain lifestyle changes. This chapter explores various factors in your lifestyle that can impact acne and provides practical strategies for promoting clearer, healthier skin.

Managing Stress: A Calm Mind for Clear Skin

Stress can trigger hormonal fluctuations that may exacerbate acne. It can also take a toll on both your mental well-being and your skin. Understanding the connection between stress and acne is a crucial step in managing and preventing breakouts. This section explores the link between stress and skin health and provides practical stress management techniques.

Managing Stress for Clearer Skin

This section explores effective stress management techniques to promote clearer and healthier skin.

1. Understanding the Stress-Acne Connection
Hormonal Impact:
Stress triggers the release of hormones such as cortisol, which can lead

to increased oil production and inflammation in the skin. This hormonal response may contribute to the development or exacerbation of acne.

Immune System Response:

Stress can also weaken the immune system, making it less effective in fighting off acne-causing bacteria. As a result, the skin becomes more susceptible to breakouts.

2. Mindfulness and Relaxation Techniques

Meditation and Mindfulness:

Incorporate mindfulness meditation into your daily routine. This practice involves focusing your attention on the present moment, which can help reduce stress and promote a sense of calm.

Deep Breathing Exercises:

Practice deep breathing exercises to activate the body's relaxation response. Deep, slow breaths can help lower cortisol levels and alleviate stress.

Progressive Muscle Relaxation:

Engage in progressive muscle relaxation, a technique that involves tensing and then slowly relaxing each muscle group. This helps release physical tension associated with stress.

3. Stress-Reducing Activities

Physical Exercise:

Regular physical activity is an effective stress reducer. Engage in activities you enjoy, such as walking, jogging, yoga, or dancing. Exercise promotes the release of endorphins, which can improve mood.

Hobbies and Creative Outlets:

Explore hobbies and creative outlets as a way to unwind. Whether it's painting, writing, gardening, or playing a musical instrument, these activities provide a positive distraction from stressors.

4. Time Management and Prioritization

Organize Your Schedule:

Implement effective time management strategies to reduce feelings of overwhelm. Prioritize tasks, break them into manageable steps, and allocate time for self-care activities.

Learn to Say No:

Recognize your limits and be willing to say no when necessary. Setting boundaries and managing your commitments can alleviate stress.

By incorporating these stress management techniques into your daily life, you can create a more supportive environment for your skin. In the following sections, we'll explore the importance of quality sleep, regular exercise, and other lifestyle factors in achieving and maintaining clearer skin.

Quality Sleep: The Skin's Nightly Repair

Quality sleep is a cornerstone of overall health, and its impact on skin health, including acne management, is significant. This section explores the relationship between sleep and skin, providing insights into the importance of quality rest and practical tips for improving your sleep routine.

1. **Importance of Sleep for Skin Health**
   Skin Repair and Regeneration:
   During sleep, the body undergoes essential processes for skin repair and regeneration. This includes the production of collagen, a protein crucial for maintaining skin elasticity and preventing premature aging.
   Hormonal Balance:
   Quality sleep helps regulate hormonal balance, including stress hormones like cortisol. Balanced hormones contribute to a more stable environment for the skin, reducing the likelihood of acne flare-ups.

2. **Creating a Sleep-Friendly Environment**
   Optimal Sleeping Conditions:
   Ensure your sleep environment is conducive to rest. Keep your bedroom

cool, dark, and quiet. Invest in a comfortable mattress and pillows to support a good night's sleep.

Establishing a Bedtime Routine:
Develop a bedtime routine to signal to your body that it's time to wind down. This may include activities such as reading, taking a warm bath, or practicing relaxation exercises.

3. Consistent Sleep Patterns

Regularity in Sleep Schedule:
Maintain a consistent sleep schedule by going to bed and waking up at the same time every day, even on weekends. This helps regulate your body's internal clock and enhances the quality of your sleep.

Limiting Screen Time:
Reduce exposure to screens, such as phones and computers, at least an hour before bedtime. The blue light emitted by screens can interfere with the production of the sleep hormone melatonin.

4. Strategies for Improved Sleep Quality

Avoiding Stimulants:
Limit the consumption of stimulants, such as caffeine and nicotine, particularly in the hours leading up to bedtime. These substances can disrupt sleep patterns.

Managing Stress Before Bed:
Incorporate relaxation techniques before bedtime to manage stress. This may include deep breathing exercises, meditation, or gentle stretching.

Prioritizing quality sleep is a powerful strategy for promoting clearer and healthier skin. In the next sections, we'll explore the benefits of regular exercise, the importance of quitting smoking, and additional lifestyle changes to support your journey to acne-free living.

Regular Exercise: Sweat for Skin Health

Engaging in regular physical activity offers numerous benefits for overall health, including the health of your skin. This section explores how exercise can positively impact skin health, providing practical insights into incorporating regular physical activity into your routine for clearer and healthier skin.

1. Benefits of Exercise for Skin Health

Improved Blood Circulation:

Exercise promotes better blood circulation, delivering oxygen and nutrients to the skin. This enhanced circulation supports skin health and can contribute to a vibrant complexion.

Stress Reduction:

Physical activity is a powerful stress reducer. Regular exercise helps lower stress hormones like cortisol, reducing the likelihood of stress-related acne breakouts.

2. Choosing Acne-Friendly Activities

Low-Impact Options:

Select exercise activities that are gentle on the skin, especially if you have acne-prone skin. Low-impact options such as walking, swimming, and cycling can provide the benefits of exercise without causing irritation.

Yoga and Pilates:

Yoga and Pilates are excellent choices for promoting flexibility, strength, and stress reduction. These practices often include mindful breathing, which can further contribute to a calm and balanced complexion.

3. Establishing a Regular Exercise Routine

Setting Realistic Goals:

Start with realistic exercise goals based on your fitness level. Gradually increase the intensity and duration of your workouts to build a sustainable routine.

Consistency is Key:

Consistency is crucial for reaping the benefits of exercise. Aim for at least 150 minutes of moderate-intensity exercise per week, such as brisk walking, or 75 minutes of vigorous-intensity exercise, such as running.

4. **Post-Exercise Skincare Routine**

Immediate Cleansing:

After exercising, promptly cleanse your skin to remove sweat, bacteria, and impurities. Use a gentle cleanser to prevent clogged pores.

Hydration:

Keep your skin hydrated post-exercise by applying a lightweight, non-comedogenic moisturizer. Proper hydration supports the skin's recovery process.

Incorporating regular exercise into your routine not only benefits your overall health but can also contribute to clearer and healthier skin.

Quitting Smoking: Clearing the Air for Clearer Skin

Certain habits, such as smoking, can have detrimental effects on your skin. Quitting these harmful habits is a crucial step in achieving and maintaining clearer and healthier skin. This section explores the impact of smoking on the skin and provides strategies for quitting.

1. **Impact of Smoking on Skin Health**

Premature Aging:

Smoking accelerates the aging process of the skin, leading to premature wrinkles and fine lines. The chemicals in tobacco smoke can damage collagen and elastin, essential proteins for skin elasticity.

Increased Acne Risk:

Smoking is associated with an increased risk of acne. The toxins in cigarette smoke can clog pores, contribute to inflammation, and impair the skin's ability to heal.

2. Benefits of Quitting Smoking for the Skin

Improved Blood Flow:

Quitting smoking leads to improved blood flow to the skin. This enhanced circulation supports the delivery of oxygen and nutrients to skin cells, promoting a healthier complexion.

Reduction in Premature Aging:

Ceasing smoking can slow down the premature aging process, allowing the skin to recover and regain some of its elasticity and resilience.

3. Strategies for Smoking Cessation

Seeking Professional Support:

Consider seeking professional support to quit smoking. Nicotine replacement therapies, counseling, and support groups can be valuable resources in the journey to becoming smoke-free.

Setting a Quit Date:

Set a specific quit date to mentally prepare for the change. Inform friends and family about your decision, creating a support network to help you through the process.

4. Skin Recovery After Quitting

Hydration and Skincare:

After quitting smoking, prioritize skincare. Hydrate your skin with a nourishing moisturizer, and consider incorporating products with antioxidants to support the recovery of damaged skin cells.

Patience in Skin Healing:

Be patient with the healing process. While quitting smoking has immediate and long-term benefits for your skin, it may take time for visible improvements to occur.

Quitting harmful habits, such as smoking, not only benefits your skin but also contributes to your overall well-being. In the next section, we'll explore the impact of environmental factors on the skin and strategies for protecting your skin from external influences.

By making these lifestyle changes, you can create a supportive environment for your skin to thrive. In the upcoming chapters, we'll delve into specific holistic approaches and over-the-counter treatments to further enhance your journey toward achieving and maintaining clear skin.

6

Holistic Approaches

Achieving clearer skin involves embracing holistic approaches that extend beyond traditional skincare routines.Holistic approaches often involve harnessing the power of nature to promote skin health. Here are some natural remedies that have shown promise in supporting clearer skin

Natural Remedies for Clearer Skin

Holistic approaches often involve incorporating natural remedies into your skincare routine. This section explores three natural remedies—tea tree oil, aloe vera, and green tea extract—that have shown promise in promoting clearer and healthier skin.

1. **Tea Tree Oil**
   Antibacterial Properties:
   Tea tree oil is renowned for its natural antibacterial and anti-inflammatory properties. These qualities make it effective in combatting acne-causing bacteria and reducing inflammation.

   Caution in Dilution:
   Due to its potency, it's crucial to dilute tea tree oil before applying it to

the skin. Mix a few drops of tea tree oil with a carrier oil, such as jojoba or coconut oil, to avoid skin irritation.

Application:

Apply the diluted tea tree oil to affected areas using a cotton swab or a clean fingertip. Start with a small amount and monitor your skin's response. If irritation occurs, discontinue use.

2. **Aloe Vera**

Anti-Inflammatory and Healing Properties:

Aloe vera is celebrated for its anti-inflammatory and wound-healing properties. It can soothe irritated skin, reduce redness, and support the healing process of acne lesions.

Fresh Aloe Gel:

Extract the gel from a fresh aloe vera leaf. Apply the gel directly to the affected areas, ensuring a thin, even layer. Leave it on for 15-20 minutes before rinsing with lukewarm water.

3. **Green Tea Extract**

Antioxidant Benefits:

Green tea extract is rich in antioxidants, particularly catechins. These antioxidants have anti-inflammatory and antimicrobial properties, potentially aiding in the management of acne.

Topical Application:

Consider using skincare products containing green tea extract or applying a cooled, brewed green tea compress to the skin. Alternatively, green tea can be consumed orally to complement its skincare benefits.

Tips for Using Natural Remedies:

1. **Patch Test**: Before applying any natural remedy to your face, perform a

patch test on a small area to ensure you don't have an allergic reaction.

2. **Consistency is the key:** Natural remedies may take time to show results. Be consistent in your application and patient with the healing process.

3. **Monitor Skin Response**: Pay attention to how your skin reacts to each remedy. If you experience irritation or discomfort, discontinue use.

4. **Consultation**: If you have existing skin conditions or concerns, consult with a dermatologist before incorporating new natural remedies into your routine.

Natural remedies can be valuable additions to your skincare regimen, but individual responses may vary. In the following sections, we'll explore Ayurvedic practices, acupuncture, and acupressure as additional holistic approaches to support clearer and healthier skin.

Ayurvedic Practices for Skin Health

Ayurveda, the ancient system of medicine from India, emphasizes a holistic approach to health and wellness. Incorporating Ayurvedic practices into your skincare routine can contribute to overall skin health. This section explores Ayurvedic principles and practices beneficial for achieving clearer and healthier skin.

1. **Dosha Analysis**:
   Ayurveda categorizes individuals into three doshas—Vata, Pitta, and Kapha—each associated with specific qualities. Understanding your dominant dosha can guide personalized skincare practices.

Vata Skin: Tends to be dry and may benefit from nourishing and hydrating skincare.

Pitta Skin:Prone to inflammation and sensitivity; cooling and calming products are recommended.

Kapha Skin: May be oily and prone to congestion; light and detoxifying skincare is suggested.

2. Herbal Supplements:

Ayurvedic herbs are often used in supplements to address imbalances within the body, which can reflect on the skin.

Neem: Known for its antibacterial and anti-inflammatory properties, neem is often used to support skin health.

Turmeric: With its potent anti-inflammatory and antioxidant properties, turmeric is beneficial for managing various skin conditions.

3. Abhyanga (Oil Massage):

Abhyanga involves massaging the body with warm, herb-infused oil. Regular abhyanga can improve circulation and nourish the skin.

Oil Selection: Choose oils based on your dosha. For example, sesame oil is often recommended for Vata, while coconut or sunflower oil may suit Pitta.

4. Ayurvedic Diet:

Ayurveda emphasizes balancing the body through diet. Consider the following dietary guidelines for skin health:

-**Warm, Nourishing Foods**: Soups, stews, and cooked vegetables can be grounding for Vata.

-**Cooling Foods**: Pitta benefits from cooling foods like cucumbers, mint, and leafy greens.

-**Spices**: Incorporate skin-friendly spices like turmeric, cumin, and coriander into your meals.

5. Mind-Body Connection:

Ayurveda recognizes the mind-body connection. Practices such as meditation and mindfulness can promote overall well-being, potentially reflecting positively on the skin.

Pranayama (Breath Control): Deep breathing exercises can help balance doshas and reduce stress, benefiting the skin.

6. Triphala for Detoxification:

Triphala, a combination of three fruits, is commonly used in Ayurveda for detoxification. It supports digestion and elimination, which can impact the clarity of the skin.

Oral Consumption: Triphala can be taken as a supplement or consumed as a tea to support internal cleansing.

Incorporating Ayurvedic practices into your skincare routine involves embracing a holistic approach that considers the interconnectedness of the body, mind, and spirit. As you explore these practices, be attentive to how your body responds, and consider consulting with an Ayurvedic practitioner for personalized guidance. In the next section, we'll delve into acupuncture and acupressure as additional holistic approaches for clearer skin.

Acupuncture and Acupressure for Clearer Skin

Acupuncture and acupressure are traditional Chinese medicine practices that involve stimulating specific points on the body to promote balance and healing. Incorporating these techniques into your skincare routine may contribute to clearer and healthier skin.

Acupuncture:

1. *Energy Flow*: Acupuncture is based on the concept of Qi, the vital energy that flows through meridians in the body. By inserting thin needles into specific acupuncture points, practitioners aim to balance the flow of Qi.

2. *Stress Reduction*: Acupuncture sessions are known for promoting relaxation and reducing stress. Stress management is crucial for maintaining clear skin, as stress can contribute to hormonal imbalances and inflammation.

3. *Blood Circulation*: Improved blood circulation resulting from acupuncture can enhance the delivery of oxygen and nutrients to skin cells. This can contribute to a healthier complexion.

4. *Consultation*: If considering acupuncture for skincare benefits, consult with a licensed acupuncturist. They can assess your overall health and tailor treatments to address specific concerns.

Acupressure:

1. *Pressure Points*: Acupressure involves applying manual pressure to specific points on the body, similar to acupuncture points. This technique can be performed using fingers, thumbs, or specialized tools.

2. *Stress Reduction*: Like acupuncture, acupressure can help reduce stress and promote relaxation. Stress management is crucial for preventing stress-related skin issues.

3. *Lymphatic Drainage*: Certain acupressure points are believed to stimulate lymphatic drainage, helping to eliminate toxins from the body. This can contribute to clearer skin.

4. *DIY Techniques*: You can learn simple acupressure techniques for self-application. These can be incorporated into your daily routine to support overall well-being.

DIY Acupressure for Facial Relaxation:

1. *Third Eye Point (GV 24.5):* Located between the eyebrows, applying gentle pressure to this point may help relieve tension and promote relaxation.

2. *Facial Beauty Point (ST 3):* Found along the cheekbone, near the nostril.

Gentle pressure on this point is believed to benefit facial complexion.

3. ***Heavenly Pillar (B 10):*** Situated on either side of the spine, at the base of the skull. Applying pressure to these points may help release tension and promote relaxation.

As with any holistic approach, individual responses to acupuncture and acupressure may vary. If you have specific skin concerns, consult with qualified practitioners to explore how these traditional Chinese medicine practices can be tailored to support your skincare goals.

Integrating these holistic approaches into your skincare journey can provide additional support for clearer and healthier skin.

7

Over-the-Counter Treatments

Over-the-counter (OTC) treatments play a significant role in managing acne and promoting clearer skin. This chapter delves into the understanding of OTC ingredients, explores various topical treatments, and discusses the role of oral supplements in achieving and maintaining optimal skin health.

Understanding OTC Ingredients

Navigating the world of over-the-counter (OTC) skincare products can be challenging with the abundance of ingredients. Understanding the key components empowers you to make informed choices tailored to your skin's needs.

1. **Benzoyl Peroxide:**
   Function:
   Benzoyl peroxide is a widely used over-the-counter (OTC) ingredient known for its effectiveness in treating acne. Its primary functions include:

1. *Antibacterial Properties*: Benzoyl peroxide is highly effective against Propionibacterium acnes, the bacteria responsible for acne. By eliminating

these bacteria, it helps prevent and treat acne breakouts.

2. *Exfoliation*: In addition to its antibacterial properties, benzoyl peroxide has mild exfoliating effects. It promotes the removal of dead skin cells, preventing them from accumulating and clogging pores.

How to Use Benzoyl Peroxide:

1. *Start with a Low Concentration*: Begin with a lower concentration (2.5% or 5%) to minimize the risk of dryness and irritation. Higher concentrations may be more effective but can also be more drying.

2. *Patch Test*: Before applying benzoyl peroxide to the entire face, perform a patch test on a small area to check for any adverse reactions.

3. *Apply a Thin Layer*: Use a small amount of benzoyl peroxide and apply a thin layer to the affected areas. Avoid excessive use, as more does not necessarily mean better results.

4. *Use Sunscreen*: Benzoyl peroxide can make the skin more sensitive to sunlight. Apply a broad-spectrum sunscreen during the day to protect your skin.

5. *Combine with a Moisturizer*: To counteract potential dryness, consider using a non-comedogenic moisturizer after applying benzoyl peroxide.

Caution and Considerations:

1. *Skin Sensitivity*: Some individuals may experience redness, dryness, or peeling when using benzoyl peroxide. If irritation persists, consider reducing the frequency of use or switching to a lower concentration.

2. *Bleaching Properties*: Benzoyl peroxide has the potential to bleach hair, fabrics, and colored clothing. Be cautious when applying it, and avoid contact with colored items.

3. *Avoid Mixing with Certain Products:* Benzoyl peroxide may interact negatively with certain products, such as those containing vitamin C or retinoids. Consult with a dermatologist if you plan to combine different skincare ingredients.

Effectiveness and Duration:

Timing: It may take several weeks to notice significant improvements. Consistent and patient use is key to seeing long-term results.

Maintenance: Once acne is under control, benzoyl peroxide can be used as part of a maintenance routine to prevent future breakouts.

Benzoyl peroxide is a valuable OTC ingredient for managing acne, but its effectiveness can vary from person to person. If you have persistent or severe acne concerns, consult with a dermatologist for personalized recommendations and potential prescription treatments.

Salicylic Acid:

Function:

Salicylic acid is a beta-hydroxy acid (BHA) widely used in skincare products, especially those targeting acne and oily skin. Its primary functions include:

1. *Exfoliation*: Salicylic acid is oil-soluble, allowing it to penetrate into the pores. It exfoliates the skin by dissolving the top layer of dead skin cells, preventing pore blockages and promoting a smoother complexion.

2. *Unclogging Pores*: By exfoliating within the pores, salicylic acid helps prevent and treat acne, particularly blackheads and whiteheads.

How to Use Salicylic Acid:

1. *Choose the Right Product*: Salicylic acid is available in various skincare products, including cleansers, toners, spot treatments, and masks. Choose a product that suits your skin type and concerns.

2. *Start Slow*: If you're new to salicylic acid, start with a lower concentration (around 0.5% to 2%) to minimize the risk of irritation.

3. *Apply a Thin Layer*: Use a small amount and apply a thin layer to the affected areas. Avoid using excessive product, as it may lead to dryness.

4. *Use Sunscreen*: Salicylic acid can increase skin sensitivity to sunlight.

Apply a broad-spectrum sunscreen during the day to protect your skin.

5. **Combine with Moisturizer**: If you experience dryness, pair salicylic acid with a non-comedogenic moisturizer to maintain skin hydration.

Caution and Considerations:

1. **Potential Dryness:** Salicylic acid can be drying, especially at higher concentrations. Monitor your skin's response, and adjust the frequency of use if needed.

2. **Not Suitable for Everyone**: Individuals with aspirin allergies should avoid salicylic acid, as it is chemically related to aspirin.

3. **Avoid Mixing with Certain Products**: Salicylic acid may interact negatively with certain products, such as those containing vitamin C or other acids. Consult with a dermatologist if you plan to combine different skincare ingredients.

Effectiveness and Duration:

Timing: Improvement in acne and skin texture may take several weeks. Consistent use is essential for long-term results.

Maintenance: Once acne is under control, salicylic acid can be incorporated into a maintenance routine to prevent new breakouts.

Salicylic acid is a versatile ingredient for managing acne and promoting clearer skin. As with any skincare product, individual responses may vary. If you have specific concerns or persistent skin issues, consulting with a dermatologist can provide personalized guidance.

Alpha Hydroxy Acids (AHAs)
Types of AHAs:

Alpha Hydroxy Acids include various naturally-derived acids, with two of the most commonly used in skincare being:

1. *Glycolic Acid*: Derived from sugarcane.
2. *Lactic Acid*: Found in milk and yogurt.

Functions:

AHAs are water-soluble acids known for their exfoliating properties and are often used to address concerns such as uneven skin tone, texture, and signs of aging.

1. *Exfoliation*: AHAs work by loosening and removing dead skin cells from the surface, promoting cell turnover.
2. *Addressing Hyperpigmentation*: By exfoliating the skin, AHAs can help reduce the appearance of dark spots and hyperpigmentation.

How to Use AHAs:
1. *Choose the Right Product:* AHAs are commonly found in various skincare products, including cleansers, toners, serums, and masks. Select a product based on your skin type and concerns.
2. *Start with Lower Concentrations:* If you're new to AHAs, begin with lower concentrations (around 5-10%) to allow your skin to adjust.
3. *Apply to Clean Skin:* Apply AHAs to clean, dry skin. Follow the product instructions regarding frequency and application.
4. *Use Sunscreen:* AHAs can increase sensitivity to sunlight. Always use a broad-spectrum sunscreen during the day to protect your skin.
5. *Combine with Moisturizer:* If dryness occurs, use a non-comedogenic moisturizer to maintain skin hydration.

Caution and Considerations:
1. *Potential Irritation*: AHAs can cause initial dryness or irritation. Start with lower concentrations, and gradually increase as your skin builds tolerance.
2. *Not Suitable for Everyone:* Individuals with sensitive skin may need to approach AHAs with caution. Patch testing is recommended.
3. *Avoid Mixing with Certain Products:* AHAs may interact negatively with

certain products, such as those containing vitamin C or other acids. Consult with a dermatologist if you plan to combine different skincare ingredients.

Effectiveness and Duration:

Timing: Improvement in skin texture and tone may take several weeks. Consistent use is essential for optimal results.

Maintenance: AHAs can be incorporated into a regular skincare routine for ongoing benefits in addressing skin concerns.

Alpha Hydroxy Acids offer effective exfoliation, making them valuable for addressing various skin concerns. As individual responses may vary, monitoring your skin's reaction and adjusting product use accordingly is crucial. If you have specific skin concerns or persistent issues, seeking advice from a dermatologist is recommended.

Sulfur:

Function:

Sulfur is a naturally occurring element with several properties that make it beneficial in skincare, particularly for addressing acne and inflammatory skin conditions.

1. *Anti-Inflammatory*: Sulfur has anti-inflammatory properties, making it effective in reducing redness and inflammation associated with acne.

2. *Mild Exfoliation:* Sulfur possesses mild exfoliating properties, helping to remove dead skin cells and prevent pore blockages.

How Sulfur is Used:

1. *Topical Treatments*: Sulfur is commonly found in topical treatments such as masks, spot treatments, and cleansers designed for acne-prone skin.

2. *Combined Formulations*: It is often combined with other ingredients like clay, salicylic acid, or benzoyl peroxide to enhance its effectiveness.

How to Use Sulfur:

1. **Choose the Right Product:** Look for skincare products that contain sulfur as a key ingredient. These may include spot treatments, masks, or cleansers.

2. *Patch Test*: Before applying sulfur-containing products to the entire face, perform a patch test on a small area to check for any adverse reactions.

3. *Follow Product Instructions:* Adhere to the recommended usage and application guidelines provided on the product. Overuse may lead to dryness or irritation.

4. *Use Sunscreen:* If using sulfur during the day, apply a broad-spectrum sunscreen to protect the skin from increased sensitivity to sunlight.

Caution and Considerations:

1. *Slight Odor*: Sulfur has a distinctive and somewhat unpleasant odor, which may be present in products containing this ingredient.

2. *Not Suitable for Everyone:* Individuals with sulfur allergies should avoid products containing sulfur. Patch testing is recommended for those with sensitive skin.

3. *Potential Drying Effect:* Excessive use of sulfur products may result in dryness. If dryness occurs, consider adjusting the frequency of use or incorporating a moisturizer into your routine.

Effectiveness and Duration:

Timing: Sulfur-containing products may take some time to show noticeable results. Consistent use is key for optimal effectiveness.

Maintenance: Sulfur can be incorporated into a regular skincare routine to manage acne and prevent new breakouts.

Sulfur is a valuable ingredient in skincare for its anti-inflammatory and exfoliating properties. As with any skincare product, individual responses may vary. If you have specific skin concerns or persistent issues, consulting with a dermatologist can provide personalized guidance.

Understanding these key ingredients allows you to select products aligned with your skin type and concerns. In the following sections, we'll explore various topical treatments and their applications for achieving clearer and healthier skin.

Topical Treatments

Topical treatments are essential components of a skincare routine, particularly for managing acne and promoting clearer skin, A variety of OTC topical treatments are available, including cleansers, spot treatments, and masks. Choosing products that suit your skin type and concerns is crucial.

1. **Cleansers**:
   Gentle Cleansing for Acne-Prone Skin:
   - Use a gentle, non-comedogenic cleanser suitable for your skin type.
   - Cleansing helps remove impurities, excess oil, and prepares the skin for other treatments.

Ingredients to Look For:
   - Cleansers containing salicylic acid or benzoyl peroxide can provide additional acne-fighting benefits.

Usage Frequency:
   - Use the cleanser morning and night, adjusting frequency based on your skin's needs.

2. **Spot Treatments:**
   Targeted Application for Acne Lesions:
   - Spot treatments contain active ingredients like benzoyl peroxide, salicylic acid, or sulfur.
   - Apply directly to acne lesions to accelerate healing.

Caution:

- Avoid overuse to prevent excessive drying or irritation.

3. **Masks:**

Clay Masks for Oil Absorption:

- Clay masks, particularly those with ingredients like kaolin or bentonite, can help absorb excess oil and unclog pores.

Application Frequency:

- Use masks 1-2 times a week to avoid over-drying the skin.

Additional Ingredients:

- Masks may contain additional ingredients like sulfur or salicylic acid for enhanced acne-fighting benefits.

Tips for Using Topical Treatments:

1. *Consistency is Key*: Be consistent in applying topical treatments. Results may take time, so patience is crucial.

2. *Patch Test:* Before applying a new product to your entire face, perform a patch test to check for any adverse reactions.

3. *Layering Products*: If using multiple topical treatments, consider layering them from thinnest to thickest consistency. For example, apply serums before moisturizers.

4. *Sun Protection*: Many topical treatments can increase skin sensitivity to sunlight. Always use a broad-spectrum sunscreen during the day.

5. *Adjust Based on Skin Response*: If you experience dryness, redness, or irritation, consider adjusting the frequency of product use or incorporating a soothing, hydrating product.

Incorporating these topical treatments into your skincare routine can contribute to managing acne and maintaining clearer skin. As with any skincare regimen, it's essential to tailor the products to your specific skin type and concerns. If you have persistent or severe acne, consulting with a dermatologist can provide personalized recommendations for an effective treatment plan.

Oral Supplements

In addition to topical treatments, certain oral supplements can play a role in supporting overall skin health and managing acne. This section explores key supplements and their potential benefits.

1. **Omega-3 Fatty Acids**:
   Anti-Inflammatory Benefits:
   - Omega-3 fatty acids, commonly found in fish oil supplements, have anti-inflammatory properties.
   - May help reduce inflammation associated with acne.

 Sources:
   - Fish oil supplements or incorporating fatty fish like salmon and mackerel into your diet.

Consultation:
   - Consult with a healthcare professional before starting omega-3 supplements, especially if you have existing health conditions or are taking medications.

2. **Zinc Supplements:**
   Regulating Oil Production:
   - Zinc is involved in oil gland function and may help regulate oil production, making it a potential supplement for acne management.

Sources:

- Zinc supplements are available, or you can increase dietary intake through foods like nuts, seeds, and whole grains.

Balance is Key:

- Avoid excessive zinc intake, as it can lead to imbalances in other minerals. Follow recommended daily allowances.

3. **Probiotics**:

Gut-Skin Connection:

- Probiotics contribute to gut health, and emerging research suggests a connection between gut health and skin conditions.
- Balancing the gut microbiome may have positive effects on the skin.

Sources:

- Probiotics are available in supplement form or in fermented foods like yogurt, kefir, and sauerkraut.

Variety of Strains:

- Choose a probiotic supplement with a variety of strains for comprehensive gut health support.

How to Incorporate Oral Supplements:

1. ***Consultation***:

- Before adding any supplements to your routine, consult with a healthcare professional, especially if you have existing health conditions or are taking medications.

2. ***Balanced Diet***:

- Whenever possible, aim to obtain essential nutrients from a balanced diet rich in fruits, vegetables, lean proteins, and whole grains.

3. ***Consistency***:

- Take supplements consistently as directed. Results may take time, and consistency is key.

4. ***Monitor for Side Effects***:

- Pay attention to how your body responds to supplements. If you experience any adverse effects, discontinue use and consult with a healthcare professional.

While oral supplements can complement your skincare routine, they should not replace a balanced diet or proper topical skincare. Individual responses to supplements vary, and professional guidance is recommended to ensure they align with your specific needs and health status. In the next chapter, we'll explore additional lifestyle practices and considerations for maintaining optimal skin health.

Note: Always perform a patch test when introducing new OTC products. If you have persistent or severe acne, consult with a dermatologist for personalized recommendations and potential prescription treatments.

8

Prescription Medications for Acne

Acne that persists despite over-the-counter treatments may require the intervention of prescription medications. In this chapter, we'll explore the importance of consulting with a dermatologist, delve into topical and oral prescription medications, and discuss potential side effects and risks associated with these treatments.

Dermatologist Consultation

Seeking a dermatologist's expertise is a crucial step in effectively addressing acne and other skin concerns. This section outlines the importance of a dermatologist consultation and what to expect during the process.

1. **When to See a Dermatologist:**
Persistent Acne: If over-the-counter treatments haven't yielded significant improvements.
Severe Acne: For cases involving nodules, cysts, or widespread inflammation.
Skin Concerns: Beyond acne, if you have other skin issues or concerns.

2. **Preparing for the Consultation:**

Medical History: Be ready to provide information about your medical history, including past and current medications, skincare routines, and any allergies.

List of Products: Bring a list of skincare products you're currently using, including over-the-counter and prescription items.

3. **During the Consultation:**

Skin Examination: The dermatologist will examine your skin, identifying the type and severity of acne lesions and any other skin conditions.

Discussion of Concerns: Share your specific concerns, such as acne triggers, lifestyle factors, or the impact of acne on your well-being.

4. **Personalized Treatment Plan:**

Tailored Recommendations: Based on the examination and discussion, the dermatologist will create a personalized treatment plan.

Prescription Medications: If necessary, the dermatologist may prescribe topical or oral medications.

5. **Follow-Up Appointments:**

Monitoring Progress: Regular follow-up appointments allow the dermatologist to monitor your progress and make adjustments to the treatment plan.

Opportunity to Ask Questions: Use follow-up appointments to address any questions or concerns you may have.

6. **Open Communication:**

Report Side Effects: If you experience any side effects from prescribed medications, report them to your dermatologist promptly.

Changes in Skin Condition: Keep your dermatologist informed about any changes in your skin condition between appointments.

7. **Lifestyle Recommendations:**

Skincare Routine: Dermatologists often provide guidance on an effective skincare routine tailored to your skin type and concerns.

Diet and Lifestyle: They may offer recommendations on dietary and lifestyle changes that can complement your acne treatment.

A dermatologist consultation is a valuable step in the journey to clearer skin. The expertise of a dermatologist ensures that your treatment plan is tailored to your specific needs, increasing the likelihood of successful outcomes. Don't hesitate to ask questions and actively participate in discussions about your skincare routine and overall well-being.

Topical Prescription Medications

Topical prescription medications play a crucial role in the management of acne, especially when over-the-counter treatments prove insufficient. This section explores common topical prescriptions and how they contribute to clearer skin.

1. **Tretinoin (Retin-A):**
   Function: A potent retinoid that promotes skin cell turnover.
   Benefits: Addresses both comedonal (non-inflammatory) and inflammatory acne lesions.
   Application: Usually applied once a day in the evening.
   Caution: Initial dryness and irritation may occur, so start with lower concentrations and gradually increase.

2. **Clindamycin/Benzoyl Peroxide Combinations:**
   Function: Combines an antibiotic (clindamycin) with an antimicrobial agent (benzoyl peroxide).
   Benefits: Controls bacteria and reduces inflammation.
   Application: Applied once or twice daily, depending on the formulation.
   Caution: Benzoyl peroxide may cause dryness, and it's essential to use

sunscreen due to increased sensitivity.

3. Adapalene:

Function: A retinoid effective in preventing new acne lesions.

Benefits: Addresses comedonal acne and helps prevent the formation of new lesions.

Application: Applied once a day, usually in the evening.

Caution: Similar to tretinoin, initial dryness and irritation may occur.

4. Other Topical Antibiotics:

Erythromycin and Clindamycin: These antibiotics are available in topical formulations and help control acne-causing bacteria.

Application: Applied once or twice daily, following dermatologist recommendations.

5. Combination Topical Therapies:

Custom Formulations: Dermatologists may prescribe custom topical formulations tailored to your specific skin needs.

Benefits: Combining different active ingredients can provide a comprehensive approach to acne management.

6. Application Guidelines:

Clean Skin: Apply topical medications to clean, dry skin.

Pea-Sized Amount: Use a pea-sized amount for each application to avoid excessive drying.

Layering: If using multiple topical medications, follow the dermatologist's guidance on the order of application.

7. Side Effects and Caution:

Dryness and Irritation: Common side effects include initial dryness and irritation. These usually improve over time.

Photosensitivity: Increased sensitivity to sunlight. Always use a broad-spectrum sunscreen during the day.

Topical prescription medications, when used under the guidance of a dermatologist, are powerful tools in the management of acne. They target various aspects of acne development, from reducing inflammation to preventing new lesions. It's essential to follow the prescribed application guidelines and report any side effects to ensure the safety and effectiveness of the treatment plan.

Oral Prescription Medications

Oral prescription medications are often recommended for individuals with moderate to severe acne or when topical treatments prove insufficient. In this section, we'll explore common oral prescriptions and their roles in managing acne.

1. **Oral Antibiotics:**
   Commonly Prescribed Antibiotics: Doxycycline, minocycline, and tetracycline.
   Mechanism of Action: Antibiotics work by reducing inflammation and controlling the bacteria associated with acne.
   Usage Duration: Typically prescribed for a limited period (e.g., several months).
   Monitoring: Regular check-ups and potential blood tests may be necessary to monitor for side effects.

2. **Isotretinoin (Accutane):**
   Indication: Reserved for severe or resistant cases of acne.
   Function: A powerful retinoid that addresses various factors contributing to acne, including oil production, inflammation, and the formation of comedones.
   Duration of Treatment: A course of isotretinoin usually lasts several months.

Monitoring: Close monitoring is essential due to potential side effects, including those affecting the liver, lipids, and pregnancy risks in females.

3. **Birth Control Pills:**

For Females: Certain oral contraceptives can be effective in managing acne in females.

Hormonal Regulation: They regulate hormones that contribute to acne development.

Consultation: Prescribed by a healthcare professional based on individual health considerations.

4. **Spironolactone**:

For Females: Often prescribed for adult females with hormonal acne.

Mechanism of Action: Acts as an anti-androgen, reducing the effects of male hormones (androgens) on the skin.

Monitoring: Regular check-ups may be necessary to assess its effectiveness and manage potential side effects.

5. **Usage Considerations:**

Consultation is Key: All oral prescriptions require consultation with a healthcare professional, considering individual health conditions and potential side effects.

Pregnancy Considerations: Certain medications, like isotretinoin, have strict guidelines due to potential risks during pregnancy. Effective contraception may be required during treatment.

6. **Side Effects and Risks:**

Common Side Effects: Side effects may include gastrointestinal upset, photosensitivity, and potential interactions with other medications.

Isotretinoin-Specific Risks: Isotretinoin carries specific risks, including dryness, mood changes, and, in rare cases, severe birth defects if used during pregnancy.

Oral prescription medications are valuable options for managing acne, especially in cases of moderate to severe or treatment-resistant acne. However, their usage comes with considerations and potential side effects, emphasizing the importance of consultation with a healthcare professional. Regular monitoring and open communication about any concerns are essential for a safe and effective treatment experience.

Potential Side Effects and Risks

While oral and topical prescription medications can be effective in treating acne, it's important to be aware of potential side effects and risks associated with these treatments. Understanding these considerations allows for informed decision-making and proactive management of any adverse effects.

1. **Common Side Effects:**
   Topical Retinoids (e.g., Tretinoin, Adapalene):
   Common Side Effects: Initial dryness, redness, and mild irritation.
   Management: Gradual introduction of the product, using a pea-sized amount, and incorporating a non-comedogenic moisturizer.

Topical Antibiotics (e.g., Clindamycin):
   Common Side Effects: Dryness, peeling, and potential photosensitivity.
   Management: Sunscreen use during the day and adjusting the frequency of application based on skin response.

Oral Antibiotics (e.g., Doxycycline, Minocycline):
   Common Side Effects: Gastrointestinal upset, potential photosensitivity.
   Management: Take with food to reduce stomach upset and use sunscreen to protect against photosensitivity.

Isotretinoin (Accutane):
   Common Side Effects: Dryness of the skin, lips, and eyes, mood changes.

Management: Lip balm, moisturizer, and regular monitoring of mood changes. Strict avoidance during pregnancy due to teratogenic effects.

2. Isotretinoin-Specific Risks:
Pregnancy Risks:

- Isotretinoin is highly teratogenic, posing a significant risk of severe birth defects if taken during pregnancy.

- Strict contraception measures are required during treatment, and regular pregnancy tests are often mandatory.

Other Risks:

- Potential effects on liver function, cholesterol levels, and vision.

- Regular monitoring, including blood tests, is crucial during isotretinoin treatment.

3. Hormonal Medications (e.g., Birth Control Pills, Spironolactone):
Common Side Effects:

- Potential hormonal fluctuations, mood changes.

- Gastrointestinal upset for some oral contraceptives.

Individual Considerations:

- Contraindicated for certain health conditions, and potential interactions with other medications.

4. Communication with Healthcare Professionals:
Reporting Side Effects:

- Any unexpected or severe side effects should be reported promptly to healthcare professionals.

Regular Monitoring:

- Regular check-ups, blood tests, and follow-up appointments are essential for monitoring the effectiveness and safety of prescription medications.

5. Individualized Care:

Consultation is Key:

- Each individual may respond differently to medications. Regular communication with healthcare professionals ensures that the treatment plan can be adjusted if needed.

Balancing Risks and Benefits:

- The decision to use prescription medications involves a balance between potential risks and the benefits of acne management. Open discussions with healthcare providers are crucial.

Being aware of potential side effects and risks associated with prescription medications is an integral part of acne management. Individual responses to medications vary, and communication with healthcare professionals allows for adjustments to the treatment plan as needed. While managing acne, prioritizing overall health and well-being is essential.

Prescription medications, when used under the guidance of a dermatologist, can be effective in managing moderate to severe acne. It's crucial to communicate openly with your dermatologist, adhere to their instructions, and attend regular check-ups to ensure the safety and effectiveness of the prescribed treatments.

9

Professional Treatments for Acne

Professional treatments offered by dermatologists or skincare professionals can be effective in addressing acne and promoting skin health. In this chapter, we'll explore common professional treatments, their mechanisms, and considerations.

Chemical Peels

Chemical peels are professional skincare treatments that involve the application of a chemical solution to the skin, causing it to exfoliate and eventually peel off. This process promotes the regeneration of new skin cells, leading to improved texture and appearance. Chemical peels can be beneficial for addressing acne and various skin concerns. Let's delve into the details of chemical peels.

1. **Types of Chemical Peels:**
   Glycolic Acid Peels:
   Derived from sugar cane, glycolic acid peels are effective for mild to moderate acne. They exfoliate the skin, unclog pores, and promote cell turnover.
   Salicylic Acid Peels:

Salicylic acid is particularly useful for acne-prone skin. It penetrates oil glands, exfoliates the skin, and helps reduce inflammation.

Trichloroacetic Acid (TCA) Peels:

TCA peels are more intense and suitable for moderate acne. They penetrate deeper into the skin, addressing both surface and medium-depth imperfections.

Jessner's Peel:

A combination of salicylic acid, lactic acid, and resorcinol, Jessner's peels are effective for addressing acne scars and hyperpigmentation.

2. Mechanism of Action:

Exfoliation: The chemical solution applied to the skin causes controlled exfoliation of the outer layer, revealing fresher, smoother skin underneath.

Stimulation of Collagen: Chemical peels stimulate the production of collagen, contributing to improved skin elasticity and texture.

3. Benefits for Acne:

Unclogging Pores: Chemical peels help remove excess oil and dead skin cells, preventing pore blockages that lead to acne.

Reducing Inflammation: Peels containing salicylic acid or other anti-inflammatory agents can reduce redness and inflammation associated with acne.

Improving Texture: By promoting the regeneration of new skin cells, chemical peels can improve the overall texture of the skin, including reducing the appearance of acne scars.

4. Considerations:

Downtime: The extent of downtime varies depending on the type and strength of the peel. Superficial peels may have minimal downtime, while deeper peels may require more recovery time.

Sun Protection: Sunscreen is crucial post-treatment to protect the skin from UV damage and maintain the results of the peel.

Multiple Sessions: For optimal results, a series of chemical peel sessions may be recommended, spaced several weeks apart.

Professional Guidance: Chemical peels should be performed by qualified skincare professionals or dermatologists to ensure safety and effectiveness.

Chemical peels offer a controlled and effective way to address acne and improve overall skin health. The choice of the peel type and strength should be based on individual skin needs and concerns. Consultation with a skincare professional is crucial to determine the most suitable approach and to ensure proper post-treatment care.

Microdermabrasion

Microdermabrasion is a non-invasive skincare procedure that uses a mechanical exfoliation method to remove the outermost layer of dead skin cells. This professional treatment is designed to improve skin texture, reduce the appearance of fine lines, and address certain skin concerns, including acne. Let's explore the details of microdermabrasion.

1. **Mechanism of Action:**
Exfoliation: Microdermabrasion involves the use of a machine that emits fine crystals or a diamond-tipped wand to gently exfoliate the skin's surface.
Vacuum Suction: Simultaneously, a vacuum suction device removes the exfoliated skin cells, promoting circulation and stimulating the production of new, healthier skin.

2. **Benefits for Acne:**
Unclogging Pores: By exfoliating the outer layer of the skin, microdermabrasion helps remove dead skin cells and unclog pores, reducing the risk of acne breakouts.
Improving Skin Texture: The procedure promotes the growth of new skin cells, leading to smoother and more even skin texture.
Reducing Hyperpigmentation: Microdermabrasion may help lighten dark

spots and hyperpigmentation left behind by acne lesions.

3. **Considerations:**

Mild Discomfort: Patients may experience mild discomfort during the procedure, described as a scratching or sandpaper-like sensation.

No Downtime: Microdermabrasion typically has minimal downtime. Patients can resume normal activities immediately after the procedure.

Multiple Sessions: For optimal results, a series of microdermabrasion sessions may be recommended, spaced several weeks apart.

Sun Protection: Following the procedure, it's crucial to use sunscreen to protect the newly exposed skin from UV damage.

4. **Post-Treatment Care:**

Gentle Skincare: After microdermabrasion, it's advisable to use gentle skincare products and avoid harsh or abrasive substances.

Moisturization: Keep the skin well-moisturized to support the healing process.

Sunscreen Use: Regular use of sunscreen is essential to prevent sun damage and maintain the results of the treatment.

5. **Suitability**:

Mild to Moderate Concerns: Microdermabrasion is suitable for individuals with mild to moderate acne concerns or those seeking a non-invasive approach to improve skin texture.

Consultation: Consultation with a skincare professional is crucial to assess individual skin needs and determine the most suitable treatment plan.

Microdermabrasion is a popular and effective professional treatment for addressing acne-related concerns and enhancing overall skin texture. It provides a non-invasive option for individuals seeking skin rejuvenation. As with any professional treatment, consultation with a skincare professional is essential to determine the appropriateness of the procedure for individual skin types and concerns.

Laser Therapy

Laser therapy is a professional skincare treatment that utilizes focused light energy to target specific skin concerns. In the context of acne management, laser therapy can be effective in reducing inflammation, targeting acne-causing bacteria, and improving overall skin tone.

1. **Mechanism of Action:**
   Selective Photothermolysis: Laser therapy works through a process called selective photothermolysis, where specific wavelengths of light are absorbed by target structures in the skin, such as blood vessels or pigmented areas.
   Targeting Acne-Causing Factors: Depending on the type of laser used, the energy may target blood vessels to reduce inflammation, penetrate the skin to destroy acne-causing bacteria, or stimulate collagen production for overall skin rejuvenation.

2. **Benefits for Acne:**
   Reducing Inflammation: Lasers that target blood vessels can help reduce redness and inflammation associated with acne.
   Bacterial Reduction: Some lasers, particularly those using blue light, can target and reduce the presence of acne-causing bacteria on the skin.
   Improving Skin Texture: Laser therapy can stimulate collagen production, leading to improved skin texture and reduced scarring.

3. **Types of Laser Therapy:**
   Ablative Lasers: Remove thin layers of skin, often used for treating acne scars.
   Non-Ablative Lasers: Stimulate collagen production without removing the outer layer of skin, suitable for overall skin rejuvenation.
   Fractional Lasers: Treats only a fraction of the skin at a time, promoting faster healing and recovery.
   Blue Light Therapy: Targets acne-causing bacteria on the skin's surface.

4. **Considerations:**

Professional Consultation: Laser therapy should be performed by qualified dermatologists or skincare professionals after a thorough assessment of individual skin characteristics and concerns.

Skin Sensitivity: Individuals with sensitive skin may experience some redness or swelling following laser treatment, but this is typically temporary.

*Sun Protection:*Post-treatment, it's crucial to use sunscreen to protect the treated skin from UV damage.

5. **Number of Sessions:**

- The number of laser therapy sessions required depends on the specific type of laser used, the severity of acne, and individual skin response.

- Multiple sessions may be recommended for optimal results.

6. **Post-Treatment Care:**

- Follow post-treatment care instructions provided by the skincare professional to optimize results and minimize potential side effects.

- Use gentle skincare products and avoid harsh or abrasive substances.

Laser therapy is a versatile and effective option for addressing various aspects of acne, from reducing inflammation to improving overall skin texture. However, its suitability depends on individual skin characteristics, and consultation with a qualified skincare professional is crucial for determining the most appropriate approach.

Cryotherapy

Cryotherapy is a professional skincare treatment that involves the use of extreme cold to address various skin concerns, including acne. This method utilizes liquid nitrogen to freeze targeted areas, promoting skin renewal and reducing specific skin issues. Let's explore the details of cryotherapy for acne.

1. Mechanism of Action:

Freezing Acne Lesions: Cryotherapy involves applying liquid nitrogen, a very cold substance, to freeze and remove targeted areas, such as acne lesions.

Promoting Skin Renewal: The freezing process triggers the shedding of damaged skin cells, promoting the growth of new, healthier skin.

2. Benefits for Acne:

Targeting Specific Lesions: Cryotherapy is effective in targeting individual acne lesions, reducing their size and inflammation.

Promoting Healing: By removing damaged skin, cryotherapy supports the natural healing process, leading to clearer skin.

Minimizing Scarring: Early intervention with cryotherapy may help minimize the risk of scarring associated with certain types of acne lesions.

3. Considerations:

Professional Application: Cryotherapy should be performed by qualified skincare professionals or dermatologists to ensure safety and precision.

Mild Discomfort: Patients may experience mild discomfort or a stinging sensation during the procedure, which is typically brief.

Redness and Swelling: Some redness and swelling are common post-treatment, but these effects are usually temporary.

4. Number of Sessions:

- The number of cryotherapy sessions required depends on the severity of acne and the individual's skin response.

- In some cases, a single session may be sufficient, while others may benefit from multiple sessions.

5. Post-Treatment Care:

- Follow post-treatment care instructions provided by the skincare professional to optimize results and minimize potential side effects.

- Use gentle skincare products and avoid harsh or abrasive substances.

- Sunscreen application is crucial to protect the treated skin from UV damage.

6. **Suitability**:

- Cryotherapy is suitable for individuals with specific acne lesions that can be targeted individually.

- Consultation with a skincare professional is essential to determine the appropriateness of cryotherapy for individual skin types and concerns.

Cryotherapy offers a targeted approach to addressing individual acne lesions and promoting skin renewal. As with any professional treatment, consultation with a skincare professional is crucial to ensure proper application and post-treatment care. Cryotherapy may be a valuable option for those seeking targeted intervention for specific acne concerns.

Considerations for Professional Treatments

1. *Consultation*:

Prior to any professional treatment, consult with a dermatologist or skincare professional to determine the most suitable approach for your skin type and concerns.

2. *Post-Treatment Care*:

Follow post-treatment care instructions provided by the professional to optimize results and minimize potential side effects.

3. *Combination Therapies*:

Professionals may recommend a combination of treatments to address different aspects of acne and improve overall skin health.

4. *Sun Protection*:

Sunscreen is crucial post-treatment to protect the skin from potential sensitivity and damage.

5. *Downtime*:

Some treatments may involve minimal downtime, while others may require recovery periods. Plan accordingly based on the selected treatment.

Professional treatments can be valuable additions to an acne management plan, especially for individuals with specific concerns or those seeking more intensive interventions. The choice of treatment should be made in consultation with a qualified professional, taking into account individual skin characteristics and preferences.

10

Dealing with Acne Scarring

Acne scarring can have a lasting impact on skin appearance, but there are preventive measures and treatment options available. In this chapter, we will explore ways to prevent acne scars and various treatment options for existing scars.

Preventing Acne Scars

Acne scars can be a lasting concern, but taking preventive measures can significantly reduce the risk of scarring. In this section, we'll explore strategies to prevent acne scars and promote overall skin health.

1. **Early and Effective Acne Management:**
   Prompt and effective management of acne is the first line of defense against scarring. The following practices can help:
   Gentle Cleansing: Use a mild cleanser to clean the skin without causing irritation.
   Topical Treatments: Incorporate topical treatments, such as retinoids or benzoyl peroxide, as advised by a dermatologist.
   Avoid Picking or Squeezing: Refrain from picking or squeezing acne lesions to prevent additional trauma to the skin.

2. **Sun Protection:**

Sun exposure can worsen the appearance of scars and increase pigmentation. Protect your skin by:

Regular Sunscreen Use: Apply a broad-spectrum sunscreen with at least SPF 30 every day, even on cloudy days.

Avoiding Tanning: Minimize sunbathing and tanning bed use, as these can contribute to skin damage.

3. **Healthy Diet and Hydration:**

A balanced diet and proper hydration support overall skin health:

Nutrient-Rich Foods: Include fruits, vegetables, whole grains, and lean proteins in your diet to provide essential nutrients for skin regeneration.

Adequate Hydration: Drink enough water to maintain skin hydration and promote optimal bodily functions.

4. **Avoiding Picking or Squeezing:**

Resist the urge to pick or squeeze acne lesions, as this can lead to more significant inflammation and scarring. Instead:

Hands-Off Approach: Let acne lesions heal naturally without interference.

Professional Extraction: If needed, consult a dermatologist for professional extraction to minimize trauma.

5. **Professional Guidance:**

Seeking advice from a dermatologist can provide personalized recommendations for preventing acne scars:

Individualized Treatment Plans: Dermatologists can create customized plans based on your skin type, acne severity, and specific concerns.

Early Intervention: Addressing acne early can prevent the development of severe lesions that are more prone to scarring.

6. **Proper Wound Care:**

If you have acne lesions that have broken open, practice proper wound care to minimize the risk of scarring:

Cleanse Gently: Use a mild cleanser to keep the area clean without causing further irritation.

Topical Antibiotics: If prescribed, use topical antibiotics to prevent infection.

7. **Minimize Friction and Irritation:**

Reducing friction and irritation can aid in preventing scars:

Avoid Harsh Scrubs: Gentle exfoliation is preferable to harsh scrubs, which can exacerbate inflammation.

Soft Fabrics: Choose soft fabrics for clothing and bedding to minimize irritation on the skin.

Preventing acne scars involves a combination of good skincare practices, sun protection, a healthy lifestyle, and, when needed, professional guidance. By taking proactive measures, individuals can significantly reduce the likelihood of developing lasting acne scars.

Treatment Options for Acne Scars

Addressing existing acne scars involves a combination of professional treatments and at-home care. In this section, we'll explore various treatment options that can help reduce the appearance of acne scars and improve overall skin texture.

1. **Laser Therapy:**

Mechanism:

- Fractional lasers stimulate collagen production, promoting skin renewal and reducing the appearance of scars.

Types:

- Ablative lasers remove thin layers of skin, suitable for treating more severe scars.

- Non-ablative lasers promote collagen production without removing the outer skin layer.

Considerations:

- Multiple sessions may be required.

- Sun protection is crucial post-treatment.

2. **Microneedling**:

Mechanism:

- Involves creating micro-injuries in the skin using a device with fine needles, triggering collagen production and improving scar texture.

Benefits:

- Can be effective for various types of scars.

- Minimal downtime.

Number of Sessions:

- Multiple sessions may be needed for optimal results.

3. **Chemical Peels:**

Mechanism:

- Medium to deep peels penetrate the skin, promoting cell turnover and improving the appearance of scars.

Types:

- Glycolic acid, salicylic acid, and TCA peels are common.

Considerations:

- Downtime varies based on peel depth.

- Sunscreen use is crucial post-treatment.

4. **Dermal Fillers:**

Mechanism:

- Injectable fillers elevate depressed scars, providing a smoother skin surface.

Benefits:

- Immediate improvement in scar appearance.

- Temporary results.

Number of Sessions:
- Periodic maintenance sessions may be needed.

5. **Microdermabrasion**:
Mechanism:
- Exfoliates the outer layer of skin, promoting renewal and improving scar texture.
Benefits:
- Suitable for mild scarring.
- Minimal downtime.
Number of Sessions:
- A series of sessions may be recommended.

6. **Topical Retinoids:**
Mechanism:
- Over-the-counter or prescription retinoids promote cell turnover, improving the appearance of scars.
Benefits:
- Can be used as part of an ongoing skincare routine.
Consistency is Key:
- Results may take time; consistent use is important.

7. **Vitamin C Serums:**
Mechanism:
- Vitamin C promotes collagen synthesis, aiding in scar repair.
Benefits:
- Suitable for daily use.
Consistency is Key:
- Regular application is important for noticeable results.

8. **Alpha Hydroxy Acids (AHAs):**
Mechanism:
- AHAs, such as glycolic acid, exfoliate the skin and reduce the visibility of

scars.

Benefits:

- Can be part of a regular skincare routine.

Consistency is Key:

- Regular use supports ongoing improvement.

9. ***Silicone Gel or Sheets***:

Mechanism:

- Applied to scars, silicone gel or sheets can help flatten and fade scars.

Benefits:

- Non-invasive and can be used at home.

Consistency is Key:

- Regular and prolonged use may be necessary.

Effective treatment of acne scars often involves a combination of professional interventions and consistent at-home care. The choice of treatment depends on the type and severity of scars. Consulting with a dermatologist can help determine the most suitable approach for individual skin needs. Consistency and patience are essential for achieving positive outcomes.

11

Building Long-Term Habits

Achieving clear and healthy skin is an ongoing journey that involves consistent habits and adjustments to your skincare routine. In this final chapter, we'll explore ways to maintain clear skin, make necessary adjustments to your skincare routine, manage relapses, and embrace your natural beauty.

Maintaining Clear Skin

Maintaining clear skin requires consistent effort and a holistic approach to skincare. In this section, we'll delve into practical tips for keeping your skin healthy and blemish-free.

1. **Consistent Skincare Routine:**
   Cleansing:
   Cleanse your face twice daily to remove dirt, oil, and impurities. Choose a gentle cleanser suitable for your skin type.
   Moisturizing:
   Use a moisturizer to keep your skin hydrated. Even if you have oily skin, a lightweight, non-comedogenic moisturizer can prevent excessive oil production.
   Targeted Treatments:

Incorporate targeted treatments, such as acne medications or anti-aging products, as recommended by your dermatologist.

Sun Protection:

Apply sunscreen with at least SPF 30 every morning, even on cloudy days. Sun protection is crucial for preventing sun damage and maintaining clear skin.

2. **Healthy Lifestyle Choices:**

Balanced Diet:

Maintain a balanced diet rich in fruits, vegetables, whole grains, and lean proteins. Nutrient-dense foods support overall skin health.

Hydration:

Drink an adequate amount of water daily to keep your skin hydrated from the inside out.

Regular Exercise:

Engage in regular exercise to promote blood circulation and oxygenate your skin. Remember to cleanse your face after workouts to prevent sweat-induced breakouts.

Stress Management:

Practice stress-reducing activities such as meditation, yoga, or deep breathing. Chronic stress can contribute to skin issues.

3. **Regular Check-ins with Dermatologist:**

Scheduled Appointments:

Schedule regular check-ins with your dermatologist to monitor your skin's health and address any emerging concerns.

Professional Guidance:

Seek professional guidance for adjustments to your skincare routine, especially during changes in season or life stages.

4. **Adequate Sleep:**

Quality Sleep:

Ensure you get enough quality sleep each night. Adequate rest supports overall well-being, including skin health.

Silk Pillowcases:

Consider using silk pillowcases, which can reduce friction on the skin and hair, minimizing the risk of breakouts.

5. Avoiding Harsh Products:

Gentle Skincare:

Avoid harsh and abrasive skincare products that can strip the skin of natural oils. Opt for gentle and non-irritating formulations.

Minimal Makeup:

If you wear makeup, choose non-comedogenic products and remove makeup thoroughly before bedtime.

6. Hygiene Practices:

Clean Makeup Brushes:

Regularly clean your makeup brushes to prevent the buildup of bacteria that can lead to breakouts.

Avoid Touching Your Face:

Minimize touching your face, as hands can transfer dirt and bacteria.

7. Stay Informed:

Skin Type Changes:

Be aware that your skin type may change over time, and your skincare routine may need adjustments accordingly.

Product Sensitivity:

Stay attentive to your skin's response to products. If you notice any irritation or sensitivity, consider switching to gentler alternatives.

Maintaining clear skin is a continuous process that involves daily habits, lifestyle choices, and professional guidance. By adopting a consistent skincare routine, making healthy lifestyle choices, and staying informed about your skin's needs, you can enjoy clear and radiant skin for the long term. Remember that individual skin types vary, so tailor your routine to what works best for you.

Adjusting Your Skincare Routine

As your skin's needs evolve with factors like age, season, and lifestyle changes, adjusting your skincare routine becomes essential for maintaining optimal skin health. In this section, we'll explore practical tips for adapting your skincare routine to meet changing requirements.

1. **Seasonal Adjustments:**
   Humidity Levels:
   During humid seasons, consider using lighter, water-based moisturizers to prevent excessive oiliness.
   Sunscreen Intensity:
   In sunnier months, you may need a higher SPF in your sunscreen to protect your skin from increased UV exposure.
   Hydration:
   In dry seasons, focus on incorporating richer moisturizers and hydrating serums to combat potential dryness.

2. **Age-Related Changes:**
   Anti-Aging Products:
   Introduce anti-aging products, such as retinoids or peptides, as your skin ages to address fine lines and maintain elasticity.
   Hydration:
   Aging skin often requires more hydration. Opt for hydrating ingredients like hyaluronic acid in your moisturizers.
   Gentler Formulations:
   Consider using gentler formulations as your skin becomes more delicate. Avoid harsh exfoliants and opt for mild options.

3. **Product Sensitivity**:

Patch Testing:

Before incorporating new products, perform patch tests to check for any adverse reactions or sensitivity.

Minimalist Approach:

- Simplify your routine if you notice signs of sensitivity. Stick to essential products and reintroduce others gradually.

4. **Adjusting for Skin Conditions:**

Acne-Prone Skin:

If you have acne-prone skin, continue using targeted treatments but adjust the frequency based on the current condition of your skin.

Sensitive Skin:

For sensitive skin, opt for fragrance-free and hypoallergenic products to minimize the risk of irritation.

5. **Personalizing Your Routine:**

Individual Needs:

Customize your routine based on your skin's individual needs. Some areas might require more hydration, while others may need targeted treatments.

Professional Guidance:

- Consult with your dermatologist for personalized advice on adjusting your routine. They can recommend specific products based on your skin type.

6. **Product Expiry:**

Check Expiration Dates:

Regularly check the expiration dates of your skincare products. Expired products may not be as effective and can even cause irritation.

Discard Old Products:

Discard any products that have changed in color, consistency, or smell, as these signs indicate potential contamination.

7. Regular Skin Assessments:

Self-Examinations:

Periodically assess your skin's condition. Look for changes in texture, hydration levels, or the appearance of new concerns.

Professional Skin Checks:

Schedule regular skin checks with your dermatologist to catch any potential issues early.

8. Listen to Your Skin:

Adjustments as Needed:

If your skin is showing signs of dryness, redness, or excessive oiliness, be ready to make adjustments promptly.

Consistency:

Despite adjustments, maintain consistency in your core routine. Consistent habits contribute to overall skin health.

Adapting your skincare routine is a proactive approach to ensuring your skin receives the care it needs at different stages and under various conditions. By staying attuned to your skin's signals, embracing a flexible approach, and seeking professional advice when necessary, you can maintain a skincare routine that nurtures healthy and radiant skin.

Recognizing and Managing Relapses

Despite your best efforts, skin issues may occasionally resurface. Recognizing and effectively managing relapses are crucial aspects of maintaining clear and healthy skin. In this section, we'll explore strategies for identifying relapses and implementing effective solutions.

1. Understanding Triggers:

Identify Potential Triggers:

Take note of factors that may trigger relapses, such as stress, dietary changes, hormonal fluctuations, or changes in skincare products.

Keep a Skincare Journal:

Maintain a skincare journal to track product usage, diet, stress levels, and any notable changes in your skin.

2. Prompt Action:

Early Intervention:

Act promptly at the first signs of a relapse. This may involve revisiting your skincare routine, adjusting products, or seeking professional advice.

Consult with Dermatologist:

If the relapse is persistent or severe, consult with your dermatologist for personalized guidance and potential adjustments to your treatment plan.

3. Reassess Your Skincare Routine:

Product Evaluation:

Evaluate your current skincare products. Check for any recent additions or changes that may be contributing to the relapse.

Simplify Routine:

Consider simplifying your routine to essential products, especially if you've introduced new products recently.

4. Addressing Acne Breakouts:

Spot Treatments:

Use targeted spot treatments for acne breakouts. Over-the-counter or prescribed treatments can help minimize the impact of individual blemishes.

Gentle Exfoliation:

Incorporate gentle exfoliation to promote cell turnover and prevent the accumulation of dead skin cells that can contribute to breakouts.

5. Lifestyle Adjustments:

Stress Management:

Implement stress management techniques, such as meditation, yoga, or deep breathing exercises.

Dietary Changes:

Assess your diet for any recent changes. A balanced and nutritious diet supports overall skin health.

6. Consistent Hydration:

Internal Hydration:

Ensure consistent internal hydration by drinking an adequate amount of water daily. Hydration plays a vital role in skin health.

External Hydration:

Maintain external hydration by using a suitable moisturizer, especially if your skin is prone to dryness.

7. Patience and Persistence:

Realistic Expectations:

Understand that achieving clear skin is an ongoing process. Results may not be immediate, so be patient with the adjustments you make.

Consistent Routine:

Stick to a consistent skincare routine, even during relapses. Consistency is key to long-term success.

8. Professional Guidance:

Dermatologist Consultation:

If relapses are recurrent or challenging to manage, schedule a consultation with your dermatologist. They can offer tailored solutions and address underlying concerns.

Recognizing and managing relapses require a proactive and adaptive approach. By understanding potential triggers, taking prompt action, and reassessing your skincare routine, you can effectively navigate and minimize the impact of relapses. Remember that skincare is a dynamic journey, and addressing challenges as they arise contributes to the overall health and resilience of your skin.

Embracing Your Natural Beauty

Beyond achieving clear skin, it's essential to foster a positive relationship with your natural beauty. This involves celebrating your unique features, cultivating self-confidence, and adopting a mindset that goes beyond external appearances. In this section, we'll explore ways to embrace and enhance your natural beauty.

1. **Confidence Beyond Skin Appearance:**
Positive Self-Talk:
Practice positive self-talk to build confidence. Focus on your strengths, accomplishments, and qualities beyond physical appearance.
Set Realistic Standards:
Set realistic standards for beauty. Understand that true beauty encompasses a combination of inner qualities, kindness, and self-expression.

2. **Celebrate Your Progress:**
Acknowledge Achievements:
Acknowledge and celebrate your skincare journey's progress. Recognize the effort you've invested in nurturing your skin.
Shift Focus:
Shift your focus from perceived imperfections to the positive changes you've made and the healthy habits you've developed.

3. **Healthy Body Image:**
Appreciate Your Body:
Appreciate your body for its functions and uniqueness. Focus on what your body can do rather than how it looks.
Avoid Comparisons:
Avoid comparing yourself to unrealistic beauty standards. Everyone's journey is unique, and comparison can undermine self-esteem.

4. **Minimal Makeup Approach:**

Let Your Skin Breathe:

Consider adopting a minimal makeup approach. Allowing your skin to breathe fosters a natural, healthy appearance.

Enhance, Don't Mask:

Use makeup to enhance your features rather than mask them. Emphasize what you love about your face.

5. **Self-Care Rituals:**

Mindful Self-Care:

Incorporate mindful self-care rituals that go beyond skincare. Engage in activities that bring joy, relaxation, and fulfillment.

Holistic Well-Being:

Prioritize holistic well-being, including mental, emotional, and physical health. A balanced lifestyle contributes to radiant overall health.

6. **Diversity in Beauty:**

Appreciate Diversity:

Appreciate the diversity of beauty. Recognize that beauty comes in various forms, and each individual's uniqueness adds to this richness.

Inclusive Media Consumption:

Consume media that promotes diverse beauty standards. Follow platforms that celebrate authenticity and inclusivity.

7. **Gratitude for Your Skin:**

Express Gratitude:

Express gratitude for your skin and its ability to adapt and renew. A positive mindset can enhance your overall sense of well-being.

Self-Compassion:

Be kind to yourself. Understand that imperfections are a natural part of being human, and self-compassion is a powerful practice.

8. **Beyond External Validation:**

Inner Fulfillment:

Seek fulfillment from within rather than relying solely on external validation. Confidence grounded in self-acceptance is enduring.

Continuous Growth:

Embrace personal growth and self-improvement. Strive for continuous development beyond appearance-based goals.

Embracing your natural beauty is an empowering journey that extends beyond skincare. By cultivating self-confidence, appreciating your unique qualities, and adopting a mindset that values holistic well-being, you can radiate beauty from within. Remember that your skin is just one aspect of your overall self, and true beauty is a reflection of your authenticity and self-love.

Building long-term habits for clear and healthy skin involves a commitment to consistent skincare, adjustments based on changing needs, and a positive mindset. Recognize that maintaining clear skin is an ongoing process, and occasional challenges are part of the journey. Embrace your natural beauty, celebrate your progress, and prioritize overall well-being. By adopting these habits, you can enjoy clear and radiant skin for the long term.

12

Positive Affirmations for Self-Love

Absolutely, fostering self-love is a wonderful practice for overall well-being. Here are some positive affirmations to inspire self-love and confidence:

1. I am worthy of love and kindness.

2. I embrace my uniqueness and celebrate my individuality.

3. My worth is not determined by my appearance; I am valuable just as I am.

4. I choose to see beauty in myself and others.

5. I am deserving of all the good things life has to offer.

6. My imperfections make me unique and special.

7. I am proud of the person I am becoming.

8. I radiate confidence, self-respect, and inner harmony.

9. I am on a journey of self-discovery, and I am learning and growing every day.

10. I am deserving of love and respect from myself and others.

11. I release any negative self-talk and embrace positive affirmations.

12. My self-worth is not dependent on the opinions of others.

13. I am grateful for my body and all that it does for me.

14. I am a work in progress, and that's perfectly okay.

15. I treat myself with kindness and understanding.

16. I trust in my ability to overcome challenges.

17. I am empowered, confident, and full of positive energy.

18. I am surrounded by love and support.

19. My heart is open, and I am ready to receive love.

20. I am enough just as I am, and I am constantly evolving into the best version of myself.

21. I am confident and beautiful in my natural skin.

22. My uniqueness is my strength, and I embrace it fully.

23. I am deserving of love and acceptance, exactly as I am.

Repeat these affirmations daily, personalize them to resonate with your own experiences, and watch how they contribute to building a positive and loving mindset.

Conclusion

Congratulations on completing this comprehensive guide to achieving clear and healthy skin! Your commitment to understanding the intricacies of skincare and adopting positive habits is a significant step toward radiant and confident skin.

In your skincare journey, remember that consistency, patience, and self-care are key. Your skin is unique, and its needs may evolve over time. By staying informed, adapting your routine when necessary, and embracing your natural beauty, you're on the path to long-term skin health.

Whether you're dealing with acne, aiming to prevent signs of aging, or simply seeking a glowing complexion, the principles outlined in this guide provide a solid foundation for a personalized and effective skincare routine.

As you continue on your skincare adventure, be kind to yourself and celebrate the progress you make. Skincare is not just about achieving clear skin; it's about nurturing a positive relationship with yourself and feeling confident in your natural beauty.

May your skin journey be filled with self-love, radiant glow, and the empowerment that comes from embracing the unique beauty that is you.

Wishing you clear, healthy, and beautiful skin on your ongoing journey!

Dr. Larry Godson

87